Essential Oils:

The Complete Guide to Achieving Stress Relief and Relaxation through Aromatherapy

I0413998

Table of Contents

Introduction

Congratulations on downloading Essential Oils: The Complete Guide to Achieving Stress Relief and Relaxation through Aromatherapy. Thank you for doing so. You will soon discover how much pleasure you can derive by preparing your own essential oil blends.

The following chapters will discuss many ways you can use essential oils along with some products you probably already have available. The enclosed guidelines will provide you with many formulas to improve daily skin care to what works best for cleaning your living spaces.

There are plenty of books on this subject on the market, thanks again for choosing this one! Every effort was made to ensure it is full of as much useful information as possible. Please enjoy!

Chapter 1: Methods and Benefits

Contents of Essential Oils

The physical properties of essential oils are derived from flowers and plants in a highly concentrated formula. The oils are the essence of the plant and used in small amounts can and can provide therapeutic benefits that have been used for centuries.

The bark, twigs, leaves, or flowers are beneficial when received through inhalation or your skin. The older methods used soaked the plants in oil and filtered the oil through a linen bag. In the olden days, it was called a linen sack.

Many essential oils have varying physical and emotional effects depending on which oil is used. The oil can create pain relief, stimulation, relaxation, and healing effects.

Apply to the skin through the use of carrier oils using these standards:

- ❖ Base: The harmonizing agent brings the blends together with lingering aromas such as anise, basil, bay laurel, beeswax, eucalyptus, ginger, vanilla, lemon, lime, orange, oakmoss, sandalwood, spearmint, tangerine, myrrh, and frankincense.
- ❖ Middle: These are the less aromatic longer-lasting, subtle fragrances such as bay, cajeput, carrot seed, fir needle, geranium, hyssop, rosemary, rosewood, tea tree, marjoram, sage, spruce, thyme, or anise seed.
- ❖ Top Note: The oils in this category are strong aromas that will usually evaporate and absorb into your skin quickly. For example, in this category, you will find basil, peppermint, lemon, and eucalyptus.

Carrier Oils and Essential Oils Ratios

The formula you would use:

1/2 ounce or 1 tablespoon carrier oil is equal (=) to 9 drops of your special essential oil.

Examples of Carrier Oils:

- ❖ Olive Oil is best used for most preparations and works best with the Extra Virgin Olive Oil (EVOO) with more minerals and vitamins.

- ❖ Coconut (cold-pressed) is rich in lauric acid and is considered to be chosen as a high-quality oil for promoting healthy hair and skin.
- ❖ Sunflower Oil is Vitamin E rich and is a great source for body oils, lotions, and excellent for massages.
- ❖ Sweet Almond Oil is odorless and absorbs rapidly. It is excellent for massage and is also full of protein as well as oleic acid which can help improve cholesterol and blood pressure levels.

Any of the vegetable, seed, or nut oils regularly used for cooking or food preparation can be used as carrier oil. However, be sure to search for unprocessed oils including those marked as organic or cold-pressed. Don't use the regular store oils which can contain petroleum residues and highly refined solvents. The unprocessed oils are also the richest in proteins, minerals, and vitamins which help nourish your skin.

Other Carrier Oils

- ❖ Apricot kernel oil is used as a facial oil which aids in rejuvenating and healing your skin cells.
- ❖ Arnica oil works well for bruising and inflammation but should be avoided on broken skin.
- ❖ Avocado oil is effective as a sunscreen and is excellent for aging or dry skin types.
- ❖ Calendula oil is a fabulous moisturizer and healer as a body oil for dry or damaged skin.
- ❖ Canola oil has a long shelf life. It is also light and odorless which is easily absorbed making it an excellent choice for massages.
- ❖ Castor oil is a bit heavier than some oils, making castor oil a superb choice as a moisturizer.

- ❖ Corn oil is loaded with minerals and vitamins and is used as medium weight oil.
- ❖ Evening primrose oil is an antioxidant which will prolong the shelf life of the product.
- ❖ Grape-seed oil is excellent massage oil. Grape-seed oil doesn't have a bold scent and dries quickly because of its high content of linoleic acid.
- ❖ Hazelnut oil is loaded with minerals, proteins, and vitamins which are an awesome combination for a facial.
- ❖ Jojoba oil can also extend the life of the product and leaves behind very little residue. It is excellent for very oily or dry skin conditions. Jojoba oil is a bit nutty and has a longer shelf-life than many of the other plant oils.
- ❖ Peanut oil is rich in proteins and vitamins and is one of the most basic aromatherapy oil.
- ❖ Safflower oil is light to medium weight oil for softening your skin.
- ❖ Sesame oil has an SPF factor of 4 and is loaded with minerals, proteins, and Vitamin E which makes it superb healer for many skin conditions.
- ❖ Soy oil high in Vitamin E and a good massage oil.
- ❖ St. John's Wort oil is excellent for inflammations of joints and muscles.
- ❖ Vitamin E also extends the shelf life of other carrier oils.
- ❖ Walnut oil is easily absorbed with medium weight and is good for your nervous system.
- ❖ Wheat germ oil is good for burns, stretch marks, and healing scars.

Why Choose Blends?

- ❖ Synergies are another term used for blends that are formulated by mixing oils with similar chemical families and therapeutic properties.
- ❖ Relax Synergy is a perfect relaxing aroma you can add into a bath, to lotion, or with the carrier oil.
- ❖ Germ Fighter Synergy will ward off cold germs and the flu. It is good as a cleaner. You can also dilute with the carrier oil for a nice massage, or you can choose to diffuse.

Blending Basics

You will need to understand the aromas you will be creating. These are a few of the blends so you can better comprehend which oils to choose before you begin your essential oil inventory.

Examples are as follows:

- ❖ Citrus: Lime, Lemon, or Orange
- ❖ Earthy: Patchouli, Vetiver, or Oakmoss
- ❖ Floral: Jasmine, Lavender, or Neroli
- ❖ Herbaceous: Basil, Marjoram, or Basil
- ❖ Medicinal: Tea Tree, Eucalyptus, or Cajuput
- ❖ Minty: Spearmint or Peppermint
- ❖ Oriental: Patchouli or Ginger
- ❖ Spicy: Cinnamon, Clove, or Nutmeg
- ❖ Woodsy: Cedar and Pine

You need to consider using oils in the same categories that will blend to provide a pleasant aroma. However, you can consider some of these blends using these classifications:

- ❖ Minty oils combine nicely with earthy, citrus, woodsy, or medicinal blends.
- ❖ Oriental or spicy oils combine with citrus, oriental, and floral oils.
- ❖ Floral oils will blend with woodsy, citrusy, or spicy oils.
- ❖ Woodsy oils blend well in all of the categories.

Take care and make your shopping list using your recipes so you don't purchase oils that may not be the types that will blend with the desired fragrance.

Other Oils You Might Need

First, consider how you plan on using your essential oils. If you want them for aromatherapy massage, in your bath or other beauty products, you would be okay to purchase the most basic oils.

- ❖ This is a brief listing of those oils and the instant uses:

- ❖ Eucalyptus is a good pain reliever for congestion and cold symptoms. A warm bath can boost your immune system. However, you must avoid using eucalyptus near the face of children and infants.
- ❖ Lavender is used in bath products, massage oils, or lotions to diffuse for balance, calmness, and relaxation. It also soothes minor burns.
- ❖ Lemon is excellent for aromatherapy, a natural cleaner, and a bath product.
- ❖ Peppermint has a cooling effect on aches, pains, and headaches. Do not use it near the face of children or infants.
- ❖ Tea Tree Oil is used as the carrier oil for skin irritations including acne. Add a few drops to shampoo for dandruff or lice.
- ❖ Sweet Orange is a good household cleaner, degreaser, bath product, and lotion. Diffuse the oil to help you to relax and stay focused.

Other Methods to Use:

- ❖ Adding Oils to Bath Water: Add several drops to the water before you get into the hot tub.
- ❖ Aromatherapy Vapor Inhalation: This is a steamy plan for better breathing. With just a few drops and a bit of steamy water, you will begin to feel better.
- ❖ Compress with the Oils: Add several drops of the chosen oil formula into some hot water. Dip your rag into the mixture. Apply it to your muscles, stomach, or forehead.
- ❖ Massage: Blend a few drops of the carrier oil into the skin.

How to Use Vital Essential Oils

Use an Emulsifier

Some of the essential oil methods will call for an emulsifier. The emulsifier is the product used to keep two ingredients from separating, such as one part of water and the other oil.

Massage Oils

Uplifting—Mental Clarity: Warm Spice Blends

For these blends use coconut, almond, or jojoba carrier oil.

- ❖ Cardamom is used to invigorate your body and mind to ease nervous tension. Apply three to four drops of the middle, warm aromatic green spice.
- ❖ Cinnamon Bark is used as a natural but potent stimulant. It is also used to help promote digestive health and antimicrobial germs. Apply five to six drops of the base as a dry and warm herbal spice.
- ❖ Coriander Seed stimulates the senses and soothes inflammation, as well as aiding in the digestion process. Apply three to four drops of the middle - spicy, woody, fruity aroma.
- ❖ Sweet Orange displays a cleansing and uplifting aroma as a top note with its fruity, citrusy spice. Apply 14 to 16 drops for a luxurious massage.

Sensuality and Emotional Well-Being: The Citrus Flower Blend

For these blends use grapeseed or olive carrier oils:

- ❖ Bergamot relieves tension and elevates your mood by using 12 to 14 drops of oil. The group is a top note with its floral, spicy, and citrus aromas.
- ❖ Clary Sage will naturally soothe the tension and elevate your mood with the middle- floral, musky, bitter-sweet aroma. Use two to three drops of oil for a massage.
- ❖ Grapefruit is secondary top note oil with its fresh, tangy, and citrus tones to help improve your skin health and promote detoxification. Use two to three drops of oil for the best results.
- ❖ Jasmine is of the middle group category with its warm and rich floral oil. You will stimulate your senses and warm your body. Use only two to three drops.
- ❖ Vanilla is a superb mood enhancer. Only four to five drops are necessary for the base of this creamy floral, sweet, and rich product.

- ❖ Ylang Ylang is known as a mood elevating and relaxing oil with the sweet, floral base. Only two to three drops will work wonders.

Relax Your Mind and Body: Sweet Dreams Massage

For these blends use the carrier oil best used is grape-seed:

- ❖ Chinese Rose: This middle is known as a spicy - sweet, floral oil that adds depth to the aroma with just two to three drops.
- ❖ Lavender Oil: This is of the middle category with its floral, sweet aromas as a powerful detoxifier. With 12 to 14 drops of oil, you will receive its anti-inflammatory features for a splendid night of sleep.
- ❖ Sandalwood is from the base oils in the light balsam, woody category. Sandalwood is a decongestant. It provides soothing—anti-inflammatory features are flowing after three to four drops are applied to your skin.
- ❖ Valerian Oil: Send anxiety away with this natural sleep aid from the base category of musky, woody and warm oils. Use six to seven drops for the ultimate sleep.

Chapter 2: Stress Reduction

Methods of Diffusion

Many of the items used for diffusion are products, you already have in your home. Use a diffuser to add a natural fragrance to your home and set the desired mood. It can help with concentration, insomnia, and help treat some ailments.

There is a product you can use in any space of your home where it needs an extra boost of freshness. It is relatively safe for everyone, even children. Only a small amount of oil can actually reach your body during the diffusion process.

Candle Diffusion

Purchase a beeswax or soy candle and let it burn for five minutes or so. Blow the candle out and add one drop of oil into the melted wax (not the wick). Relight the candle and enjoy. Use extra caution because the combination is highly flammable.

You can also purchase a candle diffuser that uses a tealight candle to heat the oil. The diffuser has an opening where a tray or bowl will fit. You can choose from many different shapes and colors to suit your décor. Usually, no electricity is needed. Always have a spare cord if your unit has a cord.

Tissue Diffusion

The aroma is easily transported to any space in your home. Add two to three drops of your favorite oil on a tissue. It can also be used if you are in an airplane or a work cubicle. However, you will not enjoy the scents over the entire room, just in the space where the tissue is located.

Lamp Ring Diffusers

Most lamp rings are made out of terracotta or brass shaped like a ring which is applied directly to the light bulb. Your aroma is gently diffused throughout the room. Be sure to follow the manufacturer's instructions. The oils can damage the bulb if not handled correctly.

Steam Diffusion

Pour two cups of boiling water into a container and add up to ten drops of your choice of oil. Enjoy this anytime, day or night. The steam will quickly enter the room but may not linger.

Electric Heat Diffusers

Larger areas are best covered with an electric unit, depending on the style and brand. The electrical units also more efficiently disperse the thicker oils such as Patchouli and Sandalwood. Alcohol can usually help dissolve any leftover residue in the unit.

Ultrasonic Diffusers

Ultrasonic waves and water diffuse the essential oils of your choice into your home or office space. You can choose from a variety of sizes and options. Some may also feature colored lights for enhancement. Their availability is becoming more common because they are so affordable. Some units can also provide humidity in the space if needed. It is important to follow the user instructions closely for the best results.

Cool Air Nebulizing Diffusers

Therapeutic benefits are optimized for a maximum impact. You can also wear a terracotta pendant neck diffuser. Anytime you want to smell a favorite aroma; it's there for you.

Two Diffusers Especially for the Holidays

Happy Holidays

What to Use:

1 drop Wintergreen

2 drops each of wild orange and white fir

Use either one of these blends on a piece of fabric or any other clever way you choose.

The Candy Store

What to Use:

2 drops each of wild orange and wintergreen essential oil

Just add the specified oils into a dark-colored glass bottle and create a special blend just for you. Experimentation is a great way to discover your favorite scents, so make the smallest amounts first before you double up on the amounts.

Diffuser Blends:

Combine the recommended drops to create your special scent:

Blend 1: 2 Bergamot| 4 each of Ylang Ylang & Clary Sage

Blend 2: 2 Vanilla | 7 Sweet Orange |1 Ylang Ylang

Blend 3: 6 Sweet Orange |1 Jasmine|3 Patchouli

Blend 4: 10 Lime |2 Ylang Ylang |1 Rose | 7 Bergamot

Blend 5: 9 Sandalwood|1 Neroli

Blend 6: 2 Scotch Pine|1 Rose |2 lemon|5 Sandalwood

Blend 7: 9 Sweet Orange|5 each of Lavender & Spearmint

Blend 8: 5 Lime |3 Sweet Orange | 1 of each – Jasmine & Cinnamon

Blend 9: 11 Lemon| 6 Bergamot | 3 Spearmint

Blend 10: 12 Patchouli| 5 drops Vanilla |1 Neroli |2 Linden Blossom

Blend 11: 1 Roman Chamomile|5 Rosemary|3 Lavender|1 Peppermint

Blend 12: 4 Bergamot |3 Sandalwood|1 Jasmine|2 Grapefruit

Blend 13: 5 Bergamot|1 Cypress |4 Lavender

Blend 14: 5 Lavender|1 Ylang Ylang |4 Rosewood

Blend 15: 2 Grapefruit|4 Bergamot| 2 each of Lemon and Ylang Ylang

Blend 16: 1 Cinnamon |3 Sweet Orange|6 Juniper

Healthy Bedtime Spray for the Monsters

Even though this is not a spray you use on your body; it classifies a spot in the bedtime aroma section. Some customers have called it the 'Shoo the Monsters Away' spray remedy.

Try this blend:

30 d. emulsifier

8 d. Orange

12 d. of each:

- ❖ Lavender
- ❖ Roman Chamomile

8-ounce bottle of room spray base

How to Mix:

Mix the oils with the emulsifier and base. Shake well.

How to Use:

Simply spray the monsters away and freshen the room. Spray a bit on the pillow for extra pleasure.

Bay Oil

A strong fragrance similar to clove oil is present with this special oil. You can use it as a massage oil or add it to a vaporizer or burner. Small amounts can produce a stimulant, whereas a larger amount of the oil can produce a sedative effect.

It is useful for these:

Depression

What to Use:

1 tbsp. of Jojoba Oil

2 d. of Bay Oil

4 d. each of:

- ❖ Black Pepper
- ❖ Bergamot Oil

Relaxation:

What to Use:

10 d. Bay Oil

1 d. Clove EO

2 to 3 d. Sweet Orange Oil

Almond Oil for the carrier oil

Stress Reduction

A study performed in 2013, indicated sniffing chamomile, lavender, and neroli is beneficial in reducing stress and anxiety.

Try this Method:

3 d. each of:

❖ Lavender
❖ Marjoram

Add to 15 ml Unscented Lotion

How to Use: Blend the mixture to ease your tightened muscles and relax your tense mind.

Have a Restful Massage

The Aphrodisiac Blend

What to Use:

2 d. Jasmine

8 d. Sandalwood

For Sore Muscles

What to Use:

5 d. Eucalyptus

4 d. Peppermint

1 d. Black Pepper

2 d. Ginger

The Stress Buster

What to Use:

3 d. Lavender

2 d. Lemon

6 d. Clary Sage

How to Prepare: Mix the chosen oils and store in a dark, air-tight glass container.

To Use: Apply using only ½ to 1 teaspoon for the massage.

Chapter 3: Ailments

Aromatherapy works well for individuals who suffer from illness, whether it is permanent or temporary.

Ailment 1: Acne, Stretch Marks, and Scars

What to Use:
3 d. Bergamot
10 d. Mandarin
6 d. each of:
   ❖ Tea Tree Oil
   ❖ Frankincense
2 ounces Jojoba
1-ounce Rosehip
4- 6-ounce glass pump bottle

How to Apply:

> Combine all of the essential oils first.
> Add the jojoba and rosehip oils.
> Shake well.

How to Use: Massage a few pumps into your skin twice daily as needed.

Keep the product out of the sunlight in a cool—dry place.

Ailment 2: Arthritis Aromatherapy

Carrier Oils: Anti-inflammatory properties are excellent using Jojoba, hemp seed, and pomegranate seed.

Blend #1

Use this formula:

10 d. each of:
- ❖ Helichrysum
- ❖ Roman Chamomile

2 fl. ounces carrier oil

Blend #2

Use this formula:

20 d. Roman Chamomile

4 d. Black Pepper

2 fluid ounces carrier oil

Directions for Use:

> Choose from either of these blends.
> Store it in a dark-colored container.
> Massage your joints with a small amount of the oil.
> Discuss the massage techniques with your physician

Ailment #3: Abdomen Pain

What to Use:

5 ml carrier oil

1 d. each of:
- ❖ Peppermint Oil
- ❖ Calendula or Chamomile Oil
- ❖ Clove Oil

How to Use: Mix all of the oils and gently massage your stomach using a repetitive—clockwise motion.

Ailment #4: Abscess Pain

These oils will make a compress:

2 d. each of:

- ❖ Chamomile EO
- ❖ Lavender EO
- ❖ Tea Tree EO

How to Use: Apply twice daily to the swollen tooth.

Ailment #5: Bad Breath

Bad breath can be a symptom of underlying problems that can stem from lodged food particles, plaque or other contributing lifestyle elements including coffee, cigarettes, and alcohol.

Use this mixture as a mouthwash:

- ❖ 5 ml. Brandy
- ❖ 4 d. Lavender Oil
- ❖ 125 ml. warm water

How to Use: After brushing and flossing, use this mixture to swish. Spit it out after you have finished rinsing your mouth.

Ailment #6: Blisters

You can receive a blister from insect stings, injury, burning, chafing or scalding. Never pierce a blister because it can become infected.

What to Use:

1 d. each:

- ❖ Tea Tree Oil or Lavender Oil
- ❖ Chamomile Oil

How to Use: Apply and pat it carefully but thoroughly.

Ailment #7: Breathing Issues:

Minor Conditions: Prepare this as a massage oil to be used around the back and chest area.

Dilute the following in 30 ml vegetable carrier oil:

3 d. Rosemary Oil

2 d. Cinnamon Oil

5 d. Nutmeg Oil

10 d. each of:

- ❖ Ginger Oil
- ❖ Eucalyptus Oil

Acute Conditions: You should use 4 drops of Hyssop or Eucalyptus oil using steam inhalation.

Chronic Conditions: Massage this mixture over the neck, back, and chest.

Dilute in 30 ml. vegetable carrier oil:

15 d. Eucalyptus Oil

10 d. each:

- ❖ Hyssop Oil
- ❖ Rosemary Oil

Ailment #8: Chapped Lips: Lip Balm

What to Use:

12 d. Citrus (Or your choice) Essential Oil

1 tbsp. each:

- ❖ Unrefined Shea Butter
- ❖ Beeswax Pellets
- ❖ Organic Coconut Oil

How to Prepare:

Method 1: Melt the coconut oil, Shea butter, and beeswax pellets.

Place everything in a double boiler (a bowl over the pan works).

Method 2: You can also put the mixture in the microwave for 30 seconds.

Stir, and heat it for another 30 seconds. Continue until all of the wax is melted.

Add the oils and blend the mixture.
Fill the containers and let them cool.

Ailment #9: Constipation

Along with constipation, comes the pain to your stomach.

What to Use:

- ❖ Blend in 30 ml. Jojoba Oil
- ❖ 15 d. Rosemary Oil
- ❖ 10 d. Lemon Oil
- ❖ 5 d. Peppermint Oil

How to Use: Use this combination of oils to gently massage your lower abdomen three times daily when needed.

Ailment #10: Ear Infections

If you are experiencing shooting pains in your ears, you could have a middle-ear infection.

You can relieve part of the pain with this mixture:

- ❖ 1 d. Clove Oil
- ❖ 5 ml. Grape-Seed Oil

How to Use: Massage around the ear and neck area.

Ailment #11: Fever Remedies

You should be drinking plenty of fluids such as mineral water or juice. Make some herbal teas with warm honey.

Try these variations for tea:

- ❖ Chamomile
- ❖ Rosemary
- ❖ Thyme
- ❖ Eucalyptus

Infuse for 7 minutes: Use 15 ml. oil in 600 ml. hot water.

Massage for the fever:

2 d. each of:

- ❖ Peppermint EO
- ❖ Eucalyptus EO
- ❖ Lavender EO

1 d. each of:

- ❖ Tea Tree EO
- ❖ Rosemary EO
- ❖ Black Pepper EO
- ❖ 15 ml. Evening Primrose Oil

How to Use: Massage the top of your hands, the soles of your feet, your temples, and back of your neck.

Ailment #12: Hair Loss

In one study, 44% of the women tested saw new hair growth using this formula:

Hair Loss Serum #1

You can try this for a change of pace if you want a unique blend of oils:

What to Use:

- ❖ 40 d. Carrot Seed
- ❖ 10 d. Lavender Oil
- ❖ 6 d. Clary Sage

4 d. each:

- ❖ Rosemary
- ❖ Roman Chamomile

1 tbsp. each of:

- ❖ Jojoba
- ❖ Sweet Almond

How to Prepare: Mix all ingredients and shake well.

How to Use: Warm the contents.
    Add several drops to your scalp.
    Let the solution remain overnight if possible.

Use this application several times each week.

Hair Loss Serum: #2

Try this for another alternative:
Almost 2 ounces Castor Oil
10 d. Rosemary EO
5 d. each of:
- ❖ Ylang-Ylang EO
- ❖ Lavender EO

2-ounce dropper bottle (dark glass is best)

How to Prepare:

Method 1: Pour most of the castor oil into the bottle and add the remaining oils. Shake. Apply and massage the mixture into the scalp each morning.

Let the mixture process for 20 minutes and wash your hair.

This product can also be applied at night.

Method 2: You can use the serum formula more often:

Use 1 teaspoon of witch hazel and almost 2 ounces of distilled water instead of castor oil.

Ailment #13: Headache

Rub peppermint on your temples and neck. Clary Sage is an excellent choice if you suffer from hormonal headaches.

Diffuse this blend of 1-2 drops of each:

Marjoram | Rosemary |Thyme | Lavender | Peppermint

Ailment #14: Insect Bites

Keep a bottle of these essential oils handy.

Try using these Oils:

- ❖ Lavender Oil
- ❖ Lemongrass Oil
- ❖ Thyme Oil
- ❖ Peppermint Oil
- ❖ Citronella Oil (especially for mosquitos)

How to Use: Apply the oil to the sting site to remove the sting. You can also use these as insect repellents.

Ailment #15: Leg Cramps

How to Prepare:

Make massage oil and rub the legs vigorously using the following:

- ❖ 3 d. Geranium Essential Oil
- ❖ 5 ml. Evening Primrose Oil

How to Use: Bend the knee as far as possible to help remove some of the cramping sensation.

Ailment #16: Lumbago

If you have ever experienced severe pain in the lumbar/lower spine, you understand how you could end up in bed with a stack of pillows under your knees to rest your back.

Massage for Lumbago:

10 ml. Evening Primrose Oil

3 d. Rosemary Oil

2 d. each of:

- ❖ Peppermint Oil
- ❖ Chamomile Oil

1 d. each of:

- ❖ Eucalyptus Oil
- ❖ Cardamom Oil

How to Use: Use three drops (total) of oregano, thyme, or rosemary oil added to a relaxing bath.

Ailment #17: Menstrual Cramps

What to Use:
1 to 2 d. each:
- ❖ Lavender Oil
- ❖ Rose Oil

1-ounce of sweet almond oil
How to Use: Massage the mixture on your abdomen for menstrual cramps.

Ailment #18: Pneumonia

What to Use: Fluid intake must be high and taking some tisanes (infusions) from Oregano, Thyme, or Eucalyptus could be used.

How to Use:
Boil for one minute.
Infuse for five to seven minutes
Add some honey for variety and have a drink.
Note: Cypress or Pine Oil can also be used as a steam inhalation process.

Ailment #19: Sore Muscles

What to Use:

- ❖ 3 d. Ylang-Ylang
- ❖ 5 d. Bay Laurel

4 d. each of:

- ❖ Eucalyptus
- ❖ Rosemary
- ❖ Add to 15 ml Carrier Oil

How to Use: Blend all of the oils—shake—and massage.

Ailment #20: Sleep Improvement:

How to Prepare: Mix the following:

- ❖ 10 d. Bay Oil
- ❖ 1 d. Clove Essential Oil
- ❖ 2 to 3 d. Sweet Orange Oil
- ❖ Almond Oil - carrier oil

How to Use: Blend and massage.

Ailment #21: Swollen Ankles

Many things could be the reason you have swollen ankles including varicose veins, arthritis, high blood pressure, or fluid retention. Resting and drinking plenty of fluids is a good start. A massage to the ankles could do the trick.

What to Use:

15 d. each:

- ❖ Cypress Oil
- ❖ Fennel Oil

How to Use: Massage from the feet to your knees for comforting relief.

Ailment #22: Throat Infection

What to Do:

Fix a cup of hot cup of water.

Add two drops of Tea Tree Oil to the cup.

Do this every two hours.

Chapter 4: Take Care of Your Body

To be more relaxed begins with a healthy and refreshed body.

Exfoliate Your Face

Your face gets a similar treatment without salt because salt is too harsh for your face. These three combinations will depend on your skin type.

For the Base:

- ❖ ½ Cup Raw Olive Oil
- ❖ 1 Cup Raw—Organic Sugar

Normal Skin: Mix 5 Drops each:
Frankincense, Ylang-Ylang, and Lavender

Oily Skin: Use 5 Drops each:
 Frankincense, Tea Tree, and Carrot Seed

Dry to Mature Skin: Mix 5 Drops each:
Geranium, Patchouli, and Frankincense Essential Oils

Special Treatments: Use 5 Drops of each of these:
Jasmine, Rose Oils, and Sacred Frankincense

How to Prepare:

Add the sugar into a large bowl. (Glass is best to use.)
Pour in the olive oil and the essential oils and blend thoroughly.
Tightly, close the container and label.

How to Use: Use weekly with a silver dollar scoop.

Original Scrub for the Body

You will need these to begin:

- ❖ 8-ounce container with a lid
- ❖ 1-ounce Sea Salt
- ❖ ½ Cup Raw Olive Oil
- ❖ 5 d. Ylang-Ylang
- ❖ 5 d. Frankincense
- ❖ 5 d. Lavender

How to Prepare:

Measure the salt and place it in a glass bowl.
Pour in the olive oil first and mix.
Blend in the essential oils last.

How to Use:
Scoop into the container and place the lid on tightly.
For a healthy skin texture, use a scoop weekly to your entire body.

Dry Skin Formula

- ❖ What You Need:
- ❖ 6 d. Sandalwood
- ❖ 2 d. Geranium

1 tsp. each:

- ❖ Camellia Oil
- ❖ Jojoba
- ❖ Sesame Oil
- ❖ 4 d. Neroli Oil
- ❖ 25 d. Carrot seed EO

How to Prepare: Blend each of the ingredients using a 1-ounce bottle.

Shake the contents well.

How to Use: Apply 4 to 6 drops of the blend twice daily to dry areas.

First Aid: Dry Skin Salve

What You Need:
- ❖ Approximately - 2 ounces raw coconut oil
  5 drops of each:

  - ❖ Lemon EO
  - ❖ Lavender EO
  - ❖ Tea Tree EO

How to Prepare:

Scoop the coconut oil in a glass dish and add the essential oils. Stir well.

Add the combination in a 1-ounce glass lotion pot.

How to Use:

Apply to the skin as needed. Store the salve in a dark—cool place.

Calming Body Butter

What You Need:

¼ cup each of:

  - ❖ Magnesium Oil
  - ❖ Avocado Oil
- ❖ ¾ cup Cocoa Butter
- ❖ 30 drops Lavender EO

How to Prepare:

Use low heat (double boiler), and place a large glass jar on the top to melt the butter.

Pour the melted mixture into a bowl to cool.

Using a regular mixer to blend and whip the solution.

Add the oils to the mixture.

Transfer to a glass jar or plastic container.

Store the calming body butter in the refrigerator for up to 90 days.

Tip: Always date your products to ensure good shelf-life.

Coconut Body Butter

What You Need:

- ❖ 4 tablespoons coconut oil
- ❖ 2/3 tablespoons Jojoba oil
- ❖ 10 drops rose essential oil
- ❖ 2/3 teaspoon cornstarch
- ❖ 1 ml. Alkanet infused oil

How to Prepare:

Pour the Jojoba oil, coconut oil, and cornstarch along with the infused oil in a bowl.

Heat the combination over a pan of water (double boiler style) until the coconut oil is melted.

Whip the components together. Let it cool down until it's room temperature.

Add the essential oil and whisk until the mixture is fluffy (resembles cake frosting).

Storage:

Use within 3 Months.

Store below 70 °F

Cellulite Coffee Scrub

While you are at it, you can use some Cypress and Grapefruit essential oils to help break up the fatty deposits close to your skin's surface.

What You Need:

- ❖ 5 drops Cypress EO

- ❖ 10 drops Grapefruit EO
- ❖ ½ cup olive oil
- ❖ 1 cup organic ground coffee

How to Prepare:

Measure and combine the coffee and olive oil in a large bowl.

Blend thoroughly and add the rest of the oils.

How to Use:

Scoop the contents into an eight-ounce glass container with a tight fitting top.

Use a silver size scoop to give your skin a workout.

Shaving Needs

Comforting Shaving Gel

What You Need:

7 drops each of:

- ❖ Lemongrass EO
- ❖ Grapefruit EO
- ❖ ¼ cup raw olive oil
- ❖ ¾ cup Aloe Vera Gel
- ❖ 8-ounce dark glass pump bottle

How to Prepare:

Add the drops to the bottle.

Pour in the Aloe Vera gel and raw olive oil last.

Close the container and shake well.

How to Use:

Enjoy when you pump it on your skin to shave!

Minty Fresh Shaving Cream

You Need:

- ❖ 1 teaspoon Castile Soap
- ❖ 3 tablespoons raw olive oil
- ❖ 7 to 8 drops of Peppermint

1/3 cup each:

- ❖ Shea Butter
- ❖ Coconut Oil

How to Prepare:

Put the butter and oil on low heat into a double boiler pot until the two fats are melted.

Pour the hot ingredients into a dish, and then the olive oil

Let the concoction cool for a few minutes and add the essential oil and Castile Soap.

Refrigerate for one hour (you want the mixture to become solid).

How to Use:

Remove from the refrigerator.

Use an immersion blender to whip the blended mixture with until it creates a whipped cream texture.

Place the contents into an 8-ounce glass container.

Use a portion of the cream for a unique, healthy shave.

Sensual After Shave

What You Need:

- ❖ Scant ½ cup
- ❖ Witch hazel
- ❖ Aloe Vera Gel
- ❖ 1 tsp. Vitamin E oil
- ❖ 2 tbsp. Jojoba oil
- ❖ 8-ounce dark glass pump

10 drops of each:

- ❖ Orange EO

❖ Sandalwood Oil

How to Prepare:

> Pour ½ cup of the aloe gel into the bottle and add the witch hazel.
> Add the Vitamin E, Jojoba oil, and essential oils.
> Close the container and shake.
> As usual, keep it in a dark—cool space.

How to Use:

Use this great product on your skin after your next close shave.

Bath Oil

What You Need:

> ❖ 2 ounces of carrier oil (Jojoba, etc.)
> ❖ 15 to 20 drops of your special blend of oils or 20 drops lavender essential oil

What to Do: Blend all of the components in a glass bottle.

How to Use: Add about ¼ of an ounce of the oil blend to your water.

Add the oil after the water is in the tub. Mix it well and enjoy.

Perfume or Body Spray

You may believe perfume and body sprays are the same, but they aren't. The amount of water used and the number of essential oils will vary. It all depends on how strong you want your product. Have you ever used someone else's perfume and it smelled different? You can now make that happen with your own unique blends.

Solid Perfume Recipe

What to Use:

- ❖ 7 drops essential oil
- ❖ ½ ounce Jojoba
- ❖ 1/8 ounce floral wax/beeswax

How to Prepare:

> Measure each of the products carefully and add the Jojoba along with your chosen wax product into a double boiler or similar container.
>
> When melted, remove it from the heat source and let it cool but not become solid.
>
> Pour in the chosen essential oil and stir.
>
> Pour your blend into the chosen container and let it cool to harden before handling.

How to Package:

> You will have about 0.625 ounces of a solid perfume that you can add to tiny plastic/glass jars or tins.

How to Use:

> Simply, use a bit on your wrists, neck, or behind your ears. Avoid using on areas where you may become exposed to sunlight.

One-Cup Body Spray:

What to Use:

10 tablespoons of alcohol

½ tablespoon each:

- ❖ Essential Oil
- ❖ Vegetable or glycerin oil

Perfume:

What to Use:

10 tbsp. alcohol

2 ½ tbsp. each
- ❖ Water
- ❖ Essential Oil

½ tablespoons glycerin or vegetable oil

How to Prepare:
Slowly mix the essential oils and alcohol.
In a separate container, blend the water and glycerin.
Combine the two.
Place in a closed container and let the fragrance rest for two weeks.

Shake it daily.

Body Spray: One-Ounce Size

Orange Blossom Body Spray

What You Need:
60 to 90 Drops - Essential Orange Oil (Adjust to your liking)
1-ounce Filtered Water
½ teaspoon vegetable glycerin

Patchouli Body Spray

What You Need:

- ❖ 1-ounce filtered water
- ❖ 1/8 tsp. Tunisian Patchouli
- ❖ ½ tsp. vegetable glycerin

How to Prepare:

Mix the ingredients of each recipe and shake well.

Shake well before using.

Basic Body Spray: Eight-Ounce Size

What You Need:

- ❖ 20 to 30 drops essential oils
- ❖ 8 ounces distilled water
- ❖ 1 tablespoon witch hazel (Vodka can be substituted)
- ❖ 8-ounce container

Fragrance for Brain Power

5 d. Rosemary
10 d. each:
- ❖ Patchouli
- ❖ Peppermint

Fragrance for Energizing Spray

15 d. of Grapefruit Oil
5 d. Lavender Oil

Fragrance for Comforting

15 d. Sweet Orange Oil
10 d. Cinnamon Leaf Oil

How to Use: Pour the water, witch hazel, and the chosen essential oil scents chosen in tightly sealed container. Shake vigorously before using the product.

Note: It is advisable to store this product in the refrigerator or use it within two weeks. Since water is used, it is important to realize the shelf-life of water since bacteria loves water. It is advisable to store the product in a dark space.

Stimulating Cologne

This is a masculine aroma that men and women will love!

What You Need:

A dark glass roll-on bottle to combine:
1 tbsp. (fractionated) Coconut Oil
3 d. each of:
- ❖ Cedarwood Essential Oil

❖ Balsam Fir Essential Oil

How to Prepare:
Pour the essential oil drops into the bottle.
Top off the bottle with coconut oil or other light carrier oil.

How to Use:
Apply to your pulse points for a refreshing smell.

Special Options

Vegetable Glycerin:

The oil and glycerin are what makes the scent of your product stick to your skin. If you add vegetable oil or glycerin to your fragrance, the final product is scented—moisturized skin. The jojoba oil is not heavy and a great choice because it won't leave a greasy feeling. Some people have used the apricot nut, almond, and olive oil—all depending on what base oil works best for you.

Options for Alcohol:

If you want to substitute rubbing alcohol for Vodka; you are making a good choice because the vodka does not have a lingering odor to interfere with your fragrance. Witch hazel can also be used since it is the same effect as alcohol.

Keep the Bugs Away

Healthy Bug Repellent Lotion Bar

Nothing is more worrisome than to be bothered by a mosquito. You can keep them away naturally without the commercial chemical products.

This are what you need:

¼ c. Organic Coconut Oil
1/8 c. Castor Oil

10 d. each of:

- ❖ Eucalyptus Oil
- ❖ Citronella Oil
- ❖ Clove Bud Essential Oil

1/3 c. each of:

- ❖ Raw Cocoa Butter
- ❖ Beeswax pell

How to Prepare:

> Put the castor oil, pellets, cocoa butter, and coconut oil in a heavy-duty saucepan over medium heat.
>
> Once all of the oil, butter, and wax are melted; remove from the burner to cool (3 to 4 minutes).
>
> Blend in the essential oils.
>
> Empty it into a preferred mold, tin or jar

Suggestion: A basic soap mold will do the trick. Be sure the container can handle the hot product. Cut the bars into chunks and place in a decorative container.

Directions for Use:

> Rub the bar between your hands to help the solution melt enough to rub gently over your exposed skin. You will receive a pleasing smell safe for your children.

Bug Spray: Procedure 1

What You Need:

Boiled or distilled water
Natural witch hazel
Choose from Clove, Lemongrass, Tea Tree, Citronella, Cajuput, Cedar, Eucalyptus, Catnip, Mint, or Lavender.
Optional: Vegetable glycerin
How to Prepare:

Fill an 8-ounce bottle half full of water.
Add the witch hazel and ½ tsp. vegetable glycerin (if used).
Add 30 to 50 drops of the chosen scent.

Note: Remember when the oils are increased, you are also increasing the aroma.

Bug Spray: Procedure 2

What You Need:

    1 tsp. Emulsifier

    4 ounces vinegar

    50 d. Eucalyptus

    25 d. each of:

        ❖ Spearmint

        ❖ Lemon

How to Prepare and Use:

    Blend the essential oils in a spray bottle with the emulsifier, and the vinegar.

    Shake well to mix.

    Spray around the baseboards to keep the bugs away.

Bug Repellent: Formula 3 for a Cold Air Diffuser

What You Need and Instructions:

1 drop of each essential oil: lemongrass |thyme |basil |eucalyptus

Plus about 70 ml of water

Combine each of the ingredients.

Chapter 5: Recipes for Household Cleaning

You can set a relaxing atmosphere in your home for almost any occasion using these resources.

Make Your Own Reed Diffuser

You can put this diffuser together in a few minutes, and it doesn't require a flame or plug.

Choose your aroma and gather the supplies:
- ❖ 1 glass jar
- ❖ Bamboo skewers/Reeds
- ❖ Light carrier oil (Jojoba or Almond)
- ❖ Chosen Essential Oils

How to Use:

Pour the carrier into the jar.

Add approximately twenty drops essential oil (per ¼ cup carrier oil).

Immerse the reeds and stir gently.

Let the reeds sit for one to two hours and flip the open, soaked ends.

When the reeds become dry, or the fragrance lessens; flip the reeds.

Air Fresheners: Add 50 drops to a four-ounce (½ cup) spray bottle. Shake the contents well, and you have your favorite scent.

Candles: If you have some unscented candles, place a few drops of your desired aroma to the candle before it is lit. You will automatically receive the benefits from the chosen flavor.

Natural Air Freshener Spray

What You Need:
- ❖ 6 tbsp. filtered water

- ❖ 1 tbsp. Vodka
- ❖ 10 to 40 d. essential Oil
- ❖ (Citrus, Peppermint, Jasmine, and Lavender)

How to Use:

> Place the alcohol and oils in a small spray bottle.
> Shake well and add the water.
> Shake before you spritz whenever you want to be energized.

Here are a few more versions using another method for sprays.

Each is three ounces:

Fresh Floral:
4 d. Frankincense oil
8 d. Juniper oil
6 d. each:
- ❖ Jasmine oil
- ❖ Rosemary oil

Energy Boost:
20 d. Lemon EO
8 d. Eucalyptus EO
2 d. each:
- ❖ Cinnamon EO
- ❖ Peppermint EO

Sweet Citrus:
10 d. Lavender EO
8 d. Sweet Orange EO
4 d. each:
- ❖ Bergamot EO
- ❖ Vanilla EO

Lavender Linen (2 Ounce Size)
1 tsp. Witch Hazel
15 to 20 drops Lavender
Almost 2 ounces distilled water

2-ounce dark spray bottle

How to Use:

> Add the lavender, witch hazel, and distilled water.
> Spray your linens and pillows for a tantalizing effect.
> Gel Air Fresheners

You will be amazed when you see how simple this really is to make. Lemon and lavender are good for serenity.

What You Need:
1 packet Knox Gelatin
¼ cup Vodka
1 to 2 d. food coloring
¾ cup water
15 d. essential oil (Grade oils are okay for this process.)

How to Prepare: Bring the water to boil in a small pan and add the gelatin pack.
Stir until it is dissolved. Allow it to cool at room temperature.
Pour into a small jar. Add the oils, vodka, coloring, and any decorative items.
Stir and place in the refrigerator until it is set.

You can have fun with this one by adding decorations in the gel. You can also add a wick to the bottom of the glass and make a gel candle.

Note: As the aroma fades—add a few more drops.

Carpet Freshener

What You Need:
10 d. Clove Bud EO
30 d. each of:
❖ Lemongrass EO

- ❖ Cinnamon Leaf EO
- ❖ Eucalyptus EO

½ cup Bicarbonate soda/Baking soda

How to Prepare:
Simply blend all of the ingredients in a wide mouth jar.
Close the lid for 24 hours.

How to Use: Add a sprinkle when the carpet needs refreshing, and leave it for 10 to 15 minutes before you vacuum away the residue.

Lemon Household Cleaner

What You Need:

8 ounces water
4 ounces distilled white vinegar
15 d. each of:
- ❖ Tea Tree Oil
- ❖ Lemon EO

Glass cleaning spray bottle

How to Use: Fill the bottle with all ingredients and mix.
Shake the contents before each cleaning spray.

Tip: It is advisable to use a glass container when possible. The citrus essential oils are highly concentrated and have acidic properties. Sometimes, it is best to store the products in class for this reason.

Natural Toilet Bowl Scrubber

What You Need:
1 cup vinegar

¾ cup Borax
½ teaspoon Tea Tree EO
5 drops Lemon EO

How to Use:
Combine all of the ingredients in a medium glass container.
Use ¼ to ½ cup in the toilet bowl. Let it sit for several minutes.
Use a brush to remove the stains.

For a Spray: You can also make it a bit thinner to use as a spray.
For a Scrub: Add ¼ cup of baking soda to the mix and use gloves to scrub the toilet.

Window or All-Purpose Cleaner

What to Use:
Equal Parts: Water and white or apple cider vinegar
10 to 15 drops orange or lemon essential oil
1 spray bottle

How to Prepare and Use:
Combine the products in a spray bottle to cut through grease and grime, and make the windows sparkle.

Quick Fixes

The Clothes Washer and Dryer:

Add one or two drops of oil into the washer (lemon and lavender are fresh smelling). Pour a bit of your chosen oil on a cloth and toss it in the dryer. It will make your clothes and the house have a wonderful smell.

Repel the Rodents:

If you have children or pets and want to use a bug repellent; essential oils are the answer. Choose a favorite fragrance and put several drops on a cotton ball or cloth and place it around your home. Rodents hate peppermint.

Smelly Shoes:

Add two to three drops of lemon oil to a rag or cotton ball, and put it in the shoe overnight to eliminate some of the odor. Geranium essential oil is pleasant for a different fragrance. You can place the oils directly in the shoes if you wish.

The Vacuum Cleaner:

Add two to three drops of your favorite—clean smelling aroma to the bag or filter of your vacuum cleaner.

Shelf Life of Products

Most essential oils will last from one to three years if they are stored in a glass jar or vial. A Cobalt or amber color is best.

The normal shelf life of the vegetable oil is approximately six months. However, it would need to be refrigerated in a closed container. It is recommended to write the purchase or prepared date on the container. The shelf life can be extended of each item if you add an antioxidant to your essential oil blends. Citrus oil only lasts from six months to one year as well.

Prevent cross-contamination by using a separate glass dropper for each of the oils. It will also make the oils more diluted if you accidentally mix the aromas. Unless you use the oil frequently, it is best to store it with its original top. The rubber dropper could pucker if it is too tight or loose.

Conclusion

Thank for making it through to the end of Essential Oils: The Complete Guide to Achieving Stress Relief and Relaxation through Aromatherapy. Let's hope it was informative and able to provide you with all of the tools you need to achieve your goals whatever they may be.

The next step is to decide which item you would enjoy creating. After you try a scent as it is described, you could try any way with a few adjustments. It is all up to your individualism.

Finally, if you found this book useful in any way, a review on Amazon is always appreciated!

Index

47

❖ Recipes for Household Cleaning

Smelly Shoes

The Vacuum Cleaner:

Description

You will surely want to own your personal copy of Essential Oils: The Complete Guide to Achieving Stress Relief and Relaxation through Aromatherapy.

Whether you're a beginner or pro, you will discover many different ways you can use essential oils. There is more in store for you as you learn how to prepare special blends of oils with products you may already have in your home.

The aromas are so enticing that you will not want to leave home. That is one of the benefits of mixing your oils. You can take them with you virtually – anywhere!

Each of the recipes will provide you with step-by-step instructions. You will learn how to make lotions, perfumes, shaving cream, and even insect repellent. But – it does not stop there – you can also learn how to prepare many cleaning products from your all-purpose cleaner to air fresheners.

Think of how much money you can save by making your own products.

Well, you know how to make this your personal copy.

Happy Mixing!

www.ingramcontent.com/pod-product-compliance
Lightning Source LLC
Chambersburg PA
CBHW071129280526
45787CB00003B/1223